KILLER FASHION

KILLER fASHION

JENNIFER WRIGHT

Andrews McMeel
PUBLISHING®

Artificial Silk

In 1932, the Archbishop of Canterbury rejoiced, "One of the main agents in the taming of the East End has been artificial silk."[1] Indeed, the invention of the mock silk fabric meant that lower-class women could dress like elegant ladies at a fraction of the price. The Archbishop of Canterbury did not mention, however, that a few of these finely attired women could potentially go fashionably up in flames. As fashion historian Alison Matthews David noted, the material, which Comte Hilaire de Chardonnet created in the 1890s, was made by turning mulberry leaves into a cellulose pulp with the addition of extremely combustible nitric acid. The combination caused multiple explosions at Chardonnet's workshop. This surely wasn't reassuring for women who might come in contact with any open flames while wearing their highly flammable artificial silk garments. Not everyone saw this as a disadvantage. One newspaper commented, "One only has to give a dress of Chardonnet silk to your mother-in-law, she approaches the fire, she burns, and you are rid of her."[2]

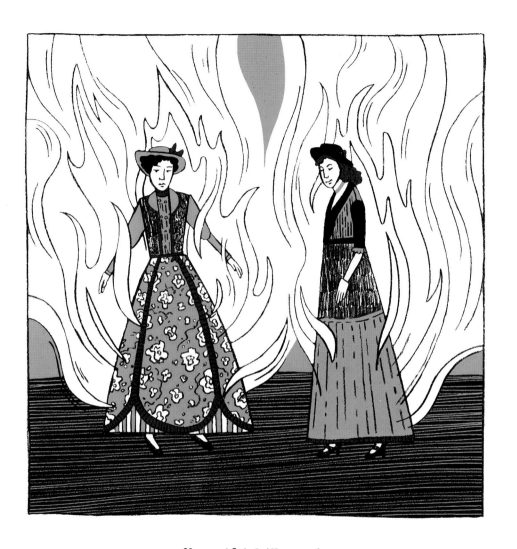

Yes, artificial silk was nice
for looking fine at half the price,
but if a candle's flame you caught,
you'd find it getting far too hot.

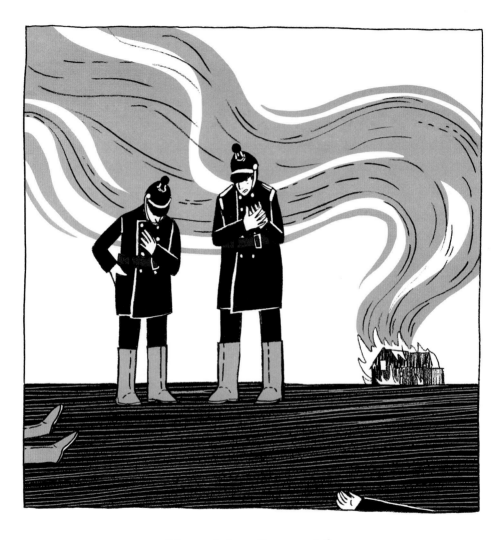

Asbestos cloth could not catch fire,
making it seem like fine attire.
But no one knew that fibers clung,
forever in their poisoned lungs.

Asbestos

Many of the clothes responsible for killing people did so because they were so flammable that the briefest of contact with any flame might transform them from garments into bonfires. But not cloth made of asbestos! Ancient Greeks and Romans admired the fire-resistant "mystical" property of this material. Marco Polo encountered it in Mongolia in 1280 and marveled at the "fabric that could not burn." [1] Emperor Charlemagne supposedly had a tablecloth made of asbestos fabric that he "cleaned" by tossing it into a fire—to the amazement of his dinner guests. [2] By the 1850s, the Paris Fire Brigade was wearing uniforms made from the material. [3] And during the Industrial Revolution, manufacturers of this fireproof fabric employed not only men, to extract asbestos from the mines, but thousands of women and children, who prepared and spun the raw fibers into cloth. [4] While these workers were not at risk from fire, they could not escape inhaling the no-less-deadly asbestos fibers. Asbestosis—scarring within the lung tissue—resulted, leading to chronic shortness of breath, increased risk of certain cancers, and, eventually, death. Unfortunately, this isn't a problem entirely confined to the past. In 2012, a woman died as a result of mesothelioma she developed from washing her husband's asbestos-covered overalls decades prior. [5]

Belladonna

Belladonna is just a prettier name for the perennial herb plant deadly nightshade. The name means "beautiful lady" in Italian [1]—in Renaissance Italy, women would use eye drops distilled from the plant to dilate their pupils. The drops made their eyes appear larger and more appealing, but there were significant downsides if you used too much. Overuse of belladonna drops could result in symptoms like blindness, swelling in the face, hallucinations, and complete delirium. One person who consumed an excess of belladonna believed they were a tailor (they weren't) and worked as a tailor might for a full day. [2] Of course, that's before patients slipped into comas, and their big eyes shut forever.

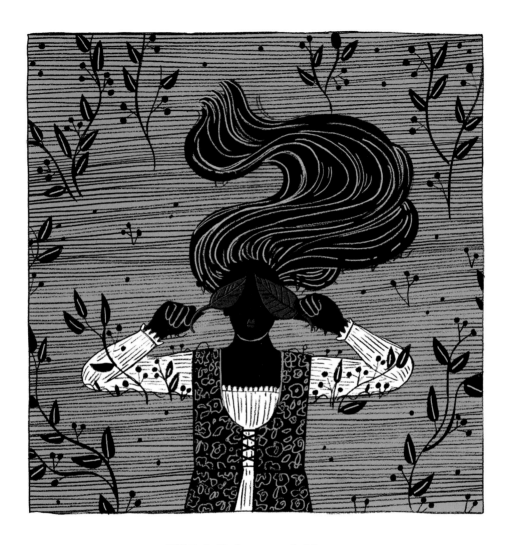

While belladonna made big eyes,
taking it was far less than wise.
For if it didn't make you blind,
it might instead just rot your mind.

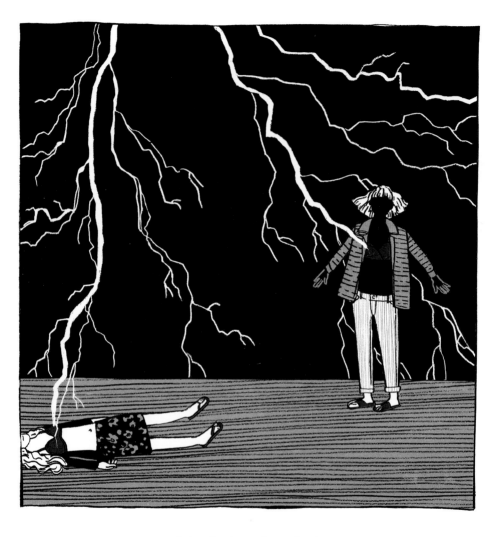

A simple piece of metal wire
holds a lady's breasts up higher.
But they can be in for quite a jolt,
if it attracts a lightning bolt.

Bras

C arrie Fisher said that for her obituary, "I want it reported that I drowned in moonlight, strangled by my own bra."[1] Which is a great funny thing to say, until you realize that *of course bras have killed people*. It's nothing to *joke* about, Carrie. In 2009, while trapped outside in a storm, two women were fatally struck by lightning. The underwire in their bras acted as a conductor and they were found dead, with burns across their chests.[2] Though, if this is making you want to go braless forever (first of all, go for it, bras are rubbish) there was another case in 2015 where a woman struck by lightning was apparently saved by her bra, as it channeled the electrical current away from her vital organs.[3]

Collars

D on't worry: The collar on your average shirt is not going to kill you. The insanely stiff starched shirt collars that dandies wore around the turn of the twentieth century, however, might. Known as a *Vatermörder*, or "father killer" in German, [1] these collars had the capacity to choke their wearer to death if he fell asleep with it still on. Such was the fate of one unlucky victim who passed out, intoxicated, on a Baltimore park bench in 1888. According to the coroner cited in *The New York Times*, "His head dropped over on his chest and then his stiff collar stopped the windpipe." [2] Even non-drinkers weren't necessarily safe. In 1912, the *Times* reported a man "suffered from an attack of indigestion which caused a slight swelling of the neck and the collar choked him to death." [3]

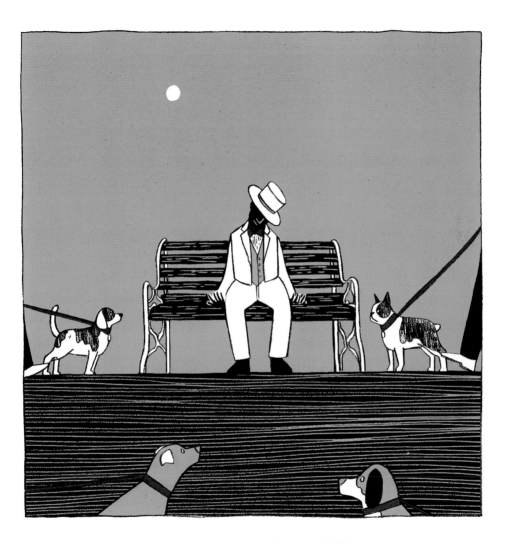

London gents spent hard-earned dollars
to buy starched detach'ble collars.
But through the night, if necks might swell,
by morning they'd be stiffs as well.

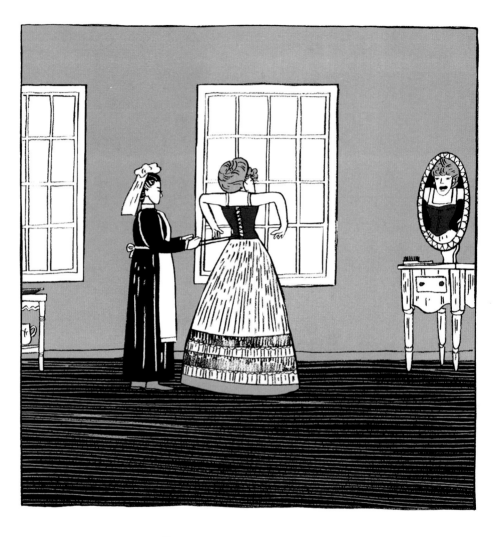

Corsets were considered a must
to cinch the waist and flatter the bust.
Victorian women held their breath,
and, stylishly, were squeezed to death.

Corsets

Simply wearing a corset isn't so bad. It's not necessarily fun, or comfortable, but it won't kill you. It's the ultratight lacing of a corset worn regularly that will cause your demise. Unfortunately, in the 1890s, women were striving to achieve the smallest waists possible. That required lacing their heavily boned corsets to what some claim was a ridiculously slimming degree. An eighteen-inch waist was considered ideal, but some girls boasted about being able to tighten their corsets (or, rather, having their strong maids tighten them) to attain sixteen- or even, in very rare cases, thirteen-inch waists. One such woman in 1859 died because the excessive tightness of her corset caused her ribs to pierce her liver. [1] Compressing a typical twenty-seven-inch waist into eighteen inches, as corsets were promised to do, is *terrible* for the body. The pressure can cause displacement of the internal organs, and habitual corset wearers could die from collapsed lungs or liver ailments. [2] And if you think those women could just stop wearing corsets, well, not so fast. Some women so distorted their ribcages with the regular wear of corsets that they could no longer stand or support the weight of their upper bodies without them. [3] Likely, no one found those poor, bent-over women particularly alluring, regardless of the waspishness of their waists.

Crinolines

At the height of "Crinolinmania" in the 1860s, four thousand crinolines—the cage-like undergarments that created fashionably full skirts—were produced a day in London. [1] If only they hadn't been! It's hard to think of an item of clothing that caused more needless death than the crinoline. They often caught fire, encircling the wearer in flames that were impossible to escape. During that time crinoline fires killed about three hundred women a year in England alone—including author Oscar Wilde's two half sisters. [2] Wearers who didn't go up in flames could be carried away by wind gusts that caught beneath their crinolines as they (ill-advisedly) walked along cliff tops. It wasn't just women who were endangered. One man was reported to have tripped over a woman's crinoline, fallen into a gutter, and was promptly run over by a carriage. Before he died, he blamed the wearer of the crinoline (though it kind of seems like he should have watched where he was walking). [3] These dangers didn't seem to deter the fans of crinolines, though. In 1861, the magazine *Littell's Living Age* lamented, "Our fair friends, when they hear of these dreadful occurrences, exclaim with the utmost sympathy, 'How *very* shocking!' But while they say so, they are wearing crinolines themselves." [4]

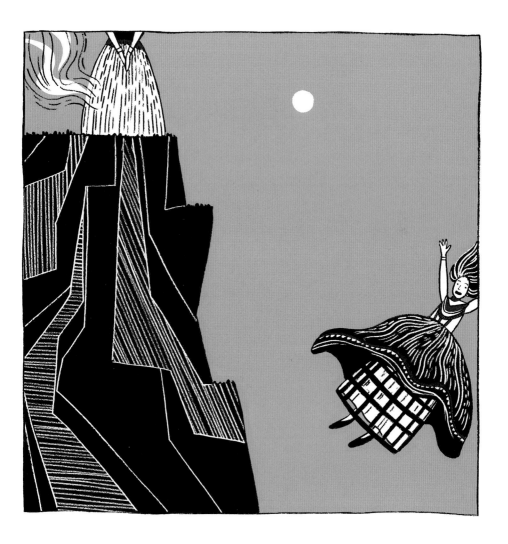

Crinoline skirts were all the rage
during the Victorian age.
But those who weren't burned up crisp
might blow aloft and fly off cliffs.

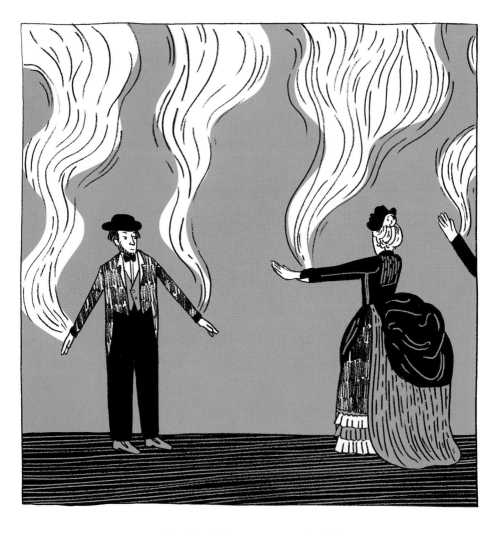

Plastic cuffs were cute and spiffy,
quick to clean up in a jiffy.
Adornments caught onlookers' gaze
'til wearers went up in a blaze.

Cuffs

Alexander Parkes invented the first man-made plastic in 1885. His creation, which he dubbed Parkesine, was thin, moldable, and easy to clean. People used it to make all manner of objects from billiard balls to brooches. [1] Those objects included decorative cuffs for their outfits. No doubt, the fact that you could easily wipe off any spots with a cloth instead of having to launder the cuffs seemed appealing. [2] Less pleasing was the fact that the material was so flammable that not only would it catch on fire if you waved it too close to a candle, but as it aged, it could also *self-ignite*. [3] They didn't last long; much though people wanted to avoid laundering their cuffs, they wanted to keep their hands more.

Felt

Being a mad hatter was not nearly as fun as *Alice in Wonderland* makes it seem. The mercury poisoning that made hat makers crazy did not, in reality, make them fun dining companions. It did give them uncontrollable twitches and tremors. It also resulted in emotional changes, mental decline, kidney trouble, respiratory failure, [1] and, regrettably, very few tea parties. Mercury poisoning, or "mad hatter disease," affected many hatmakers during Lewis Carroll's time because the mercuric nitrate that was used to make felt was exceedingly toxic. Breathing in mercury fumes all day had a deleterious effect on the hatters' health. People knew about these ill effects as early as 1757, when French doctor Jacques-René Tenon noted that most hatters did not live past age fifty and were in ill health before their deaths. In 1776, the French medical journal *Gazette de santé* described the use of mercury to produce felt as "unnecessary, bizarre, and abusive." [2] Despite the medical warnings against its use, mercury was never officially banned in England and continued being used in hatmaking until fairly recently. Had felt hats not largely fallen out of fashion by the 1960s, [3] hatmakers may have continued to be poisoned by mercury.

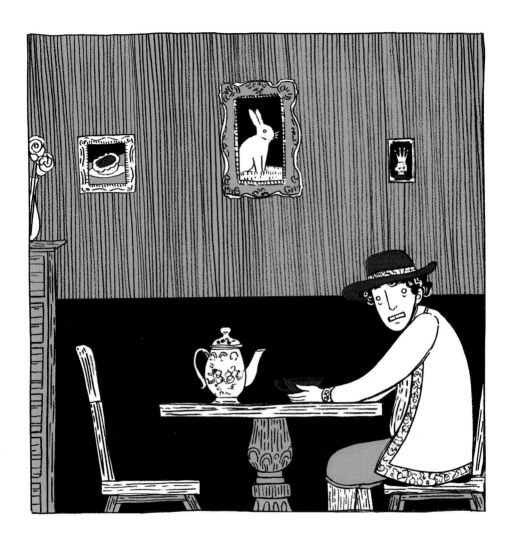

Hatters who made caps for the head
did not know they might soon be dead.
The mercury that stretched brims wide
would rot the brain that was inside.

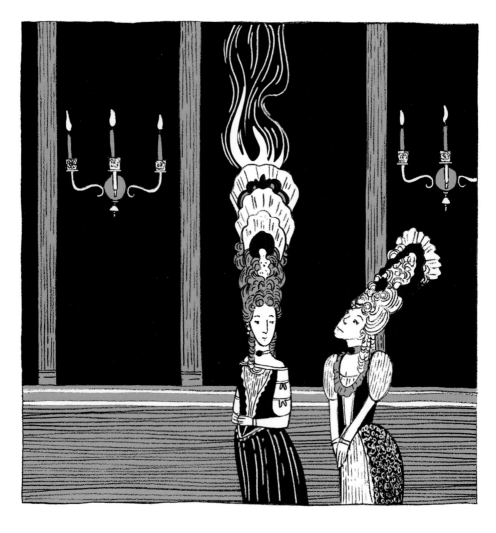

Atop their heads ladies would wear
ribbons and baubles everywhere.
But those ornaments they affixed
turned all their heads to candle wicks.

Fontange

The fontange hairdo began as an accident—and contributed to many more. It originated when Louis XIV's mistress, the Duchesse de Fontanges, fell off her horse while they were hunting. She was unharmed, but her hairdo was destroyed. So she took off a garter and tied her hair up atop her head. [1] The King loved it. However, what started out as a simple topknot soon turned into a bird's nest of lace, ribbons, baubles, and various fabrics as others began imitating Fontanges' signature 'do. Eventually, the hairstyles piled so high that—you guessed it—women began catching fire when they came too close to candles. In her book *Fashionably Fatal*, Summer Strevens recounts a letter about the unhappy fate of a Lady von Ilten in 1711: "There is no news here but that good Mrs von Ilten has burnt neck, face and hands; her fontange caught fire, she stared and fell and did not think to throw it off." Sadly, Lady Von Ilten did not survive her scorched ribbons and face. [2]

Hair Dye

The 1920s "Blonde Bombshell" Jean Harlow used to say that, if not for her hair, "Hollywood wouldn't know I'm alive." [1] Her trademark platinum hair did help her stand out at a time when black and white film had difficulty registering light. [2] Unfortunately, it probably also helped kill her. The hair dye she applied weekly was made out of Clorox bleach and ammonia. *The Atlantic* notes that this combination "produces noxious gas, hydrochloric acid, and apparently, a star-worthy shade of blonde." [3] The star-worthy shade of blonde didn't last for long. Harlow's hair began falling out by the time she was twenty-four. And though the dye created a stunningly stylish effect, it's thought to have taken a tremendous toll on Harlow, who was already in poor health. Harlow died at twenty-six from kidney failure due to a build-up of toxins in her system, which was likely linked to her frequent use of the noxious hair dye.

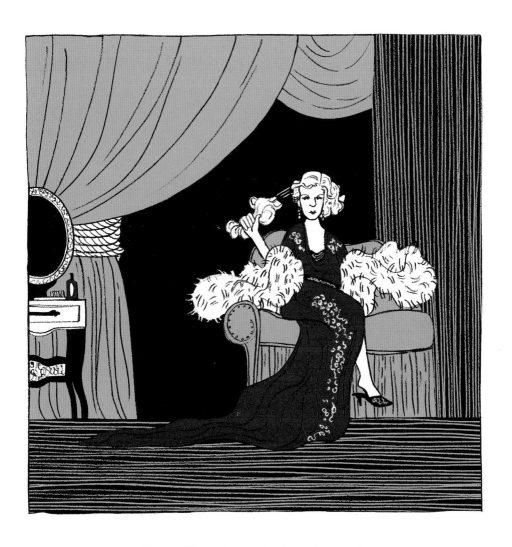

Blonde Jean Harlow had much more fun
than, truly, almost anyone.
But the head that made people stare
would soon be done with all its care.

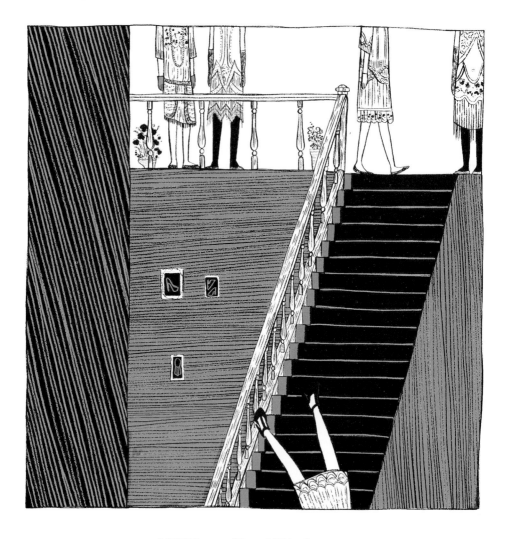

Old Winston Churchill had a mum
who thought that flats were very dumb.
Tripped on her heels, fell down the stairs,
now no one looks at what she wears.

High Heels

igh heels were always supposed to be deadly; they just weren't supposed to kill the person wearing them. Originally worn by male equestrians in fifteenth-century Persia, the shoes' heels were intended to make it easier for riders to stand up in their stirrups and shoot arrows at their enemies while galloping on horseback. [1] Male Europeans soon started wearing them as the kind of height-enhancing, intimidating accessory that also made it easier to cross over puddles or through horse manure without muddying their outfits. Fifteenth-century Italian noblewomen and courtesans then got in on the trend, and at that point, high heels became somewhat less practical. The chopines they wore could tower over a foot high. The additional height meant that the woman's family—or she herself—was wealthy enough to pay for longer skirts. [2] Chopines proved to be better for standing out than walking about. But with a somewhat shorter base, heels remained a favorite accessory of unconventional women such as Brooklyn-born Jennie Jerome, statesman Winston Churchill's mother. But the famously beautiful and stylish aristocrat became a victim of her own great taste. In 1921, while wearing a brand-new pair of high heels, she slipped down a flight of stairs, falling to her death. [3]

Lead Makeup

While white lead-based makeup was used as a kind of precursor to foundation as early as ancient Greece, its popularity soared when Queen Elizabeth I of England started using it after she contracted smallpox and was left with the disease's disfiguring pockmarks. [1] She wasn't the only one to appreciate how the makeup hid skin flaws. Unfortunately, lead poisoning caused by makeup would lead to the death of Queen Elizabeth I and many others. In 1760, Maria Gunning, the countess of Coventry, became known as a "victim of cosmetics." [2] Infamous courtesan Kitty Fisher suffered the same fate in 1767. [3] Before dying, those with poisoning from lead-based makeup experienced terrible symptoms, including hair loss, skin welts, and inflammation of the eyes. [4] Provided they kept applying the makeup, though, their skin looked ethereally pale right up until they were laid in their graves.

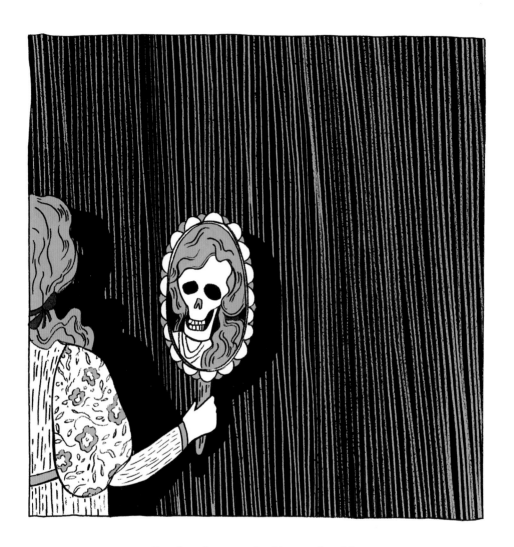

Lead makeup made skin pearly white
and turned gray faces oh so bright.
Of their complexion folks would boast
'til they became the palest ghosts.

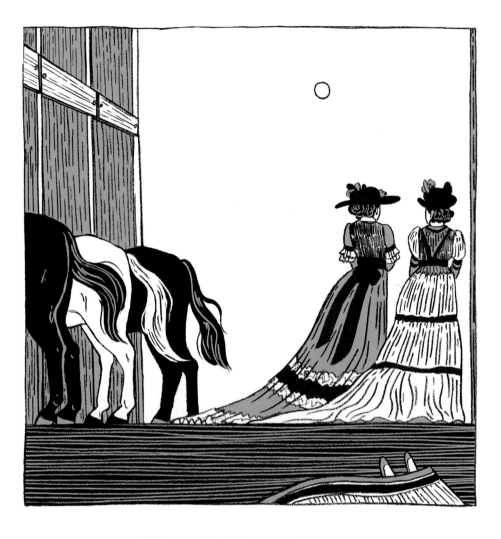

When trailing skirts were all the rage,
a sweeping hem turned coprophage.
Streets were full of animal crap,
and typhus brought eternal nap.

Long Skirts

Today, it's probably common sense that you shouldn't drag your outfit through piles of horse dung, but not so much in the 1900s. Long trailing skirts were a fashion necessity, as was walking around the city. Unfortunately, streets were covered with both horse and dog feces, as well as spit from phlegmy city dwellers. As one doctor noted in a 1900 issue of the medical journal *The Lancet*, "Women sweep the streets with the skirts of their gowns . . . and bear with them wherever they go the abominable filth." [1] Doctors observed "deadly bacilli" [2] on the hems of such skirts, which could lead to typhoid fever or consumption. Naturally, when women began wearing shorter skirts, magazines like *Harper's* wondered, "What of women's mission to be lovely?" [3] In a world where there's apparently no right way to wear a skirt, it's still probably in your best interest not to wear one covered in fecal matter.

Lotus Feet

From 850 AD to the mid-1800s, the ideal female foot in China was about four (Western) inches long. Such feet were known as "golden lotuses" and fit into special shoes. [1] No adult woman has ever had a natural foot that is four inches long, so to create these "golden lotuses," girls as young as age five would have their feet broken and then bound to prevent them from growing any larger. Their broken toes would curl beneath their feet. This maiming could lead to horrific infection if, as was not uncommon, a toenail began cutting into the flesh. Some women died from septic shock; others just lost a toe or two. But losing a toe wasn't necessarily seen as a negative, as it allowed for tighter binding and even smaller feet. [2] Unchecked infection and loss of extremities, on the other hand, are negative in terms of remaining alive. If women survived this procedure and grew to adulthood, they were left with a halting gait from walking on their heels. This gait was thought to be extremely desirable and led to better marriage prospects for women whose feet were bound. And lest you think this was a trend confined only to the ancient past, the last factory producing "lotus shoes" didn't close until 1999. [3]

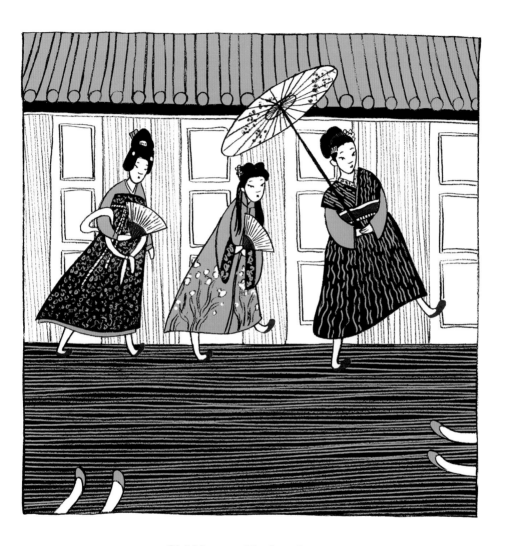

Girls' bent and broken tiny toes
were said to beckon many beaus.
But though they made a dainty walk,
they could cause deadly septic shock.

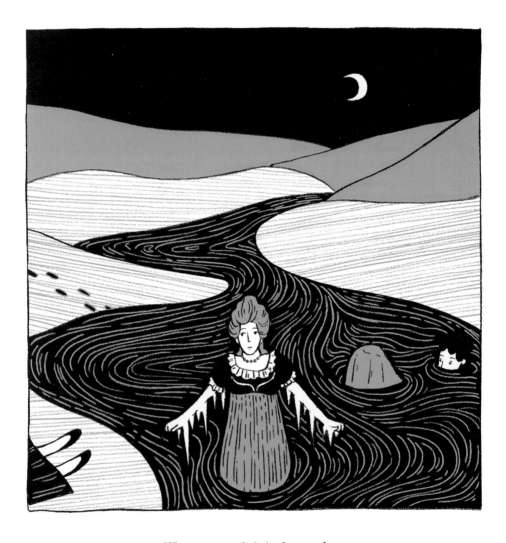

Women wetted their dresses down
to show the form beneath the gown.
And the effect was very bold—
at least until they died of cold.

Muslin

The light muslin dresses of the Directoire period in late 1700s France must have seemed like a welcome reprieve from the constraining garments women had been used to wearing. Post-Revolutionary women were expected to be liberated—in both their attitudes and their clothing. Their fashionable airy gowns were inspired by ancient Rome and Greece and were tailored to move with the body's natural form. That meant no more corsets! But, unfortunately, still some death. Women were so eager to show off their figures that some wetted their dresses to make them cling alluringly. [1] And while damp gowns might have been fine in warmer climates—like those of Italy or Greece—the French winter was less forgiving. [2] Wandering around in the snow in a skimpy, soaked dress and sandals didn't bode well for health. No wonder that an influenza epidemic struck in 1803 and was nicknamed "muslin disease." [3]

Neckties

While many fashionable accoutrements have been relegated to the past, the necktie lives on. And as it lives, it kills. The most common male accessory doubles as a noose on a not infrequent basis. As recently as 2016, Manhattan saw a "savage necktie murder of a rich globetrotting widower."[1] In 2014, a Houston man was found strangled "with a deadly weapon, namely a necktie."[2] And in 2009, a man in Wisconsin used a necktie to strangle his stepson.[3] So, keep neckties around so you can look professional for work if you must. Just realize that they can also be used to put an end to your career—*and your life.*

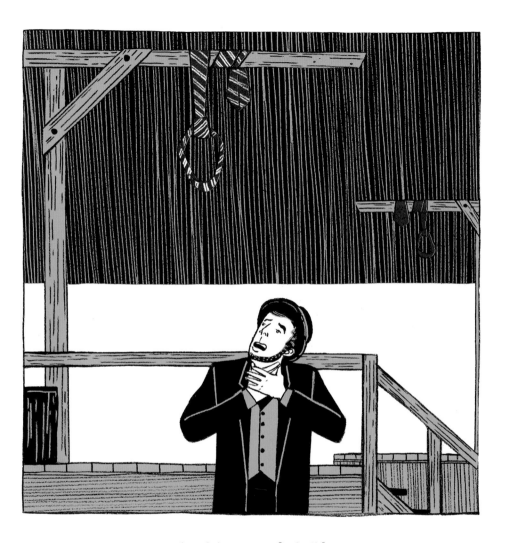

A necktie gets you far in life;
you'll look as sharp as any knife.
But be sure to wear it loose
unless you want a dandy noose.

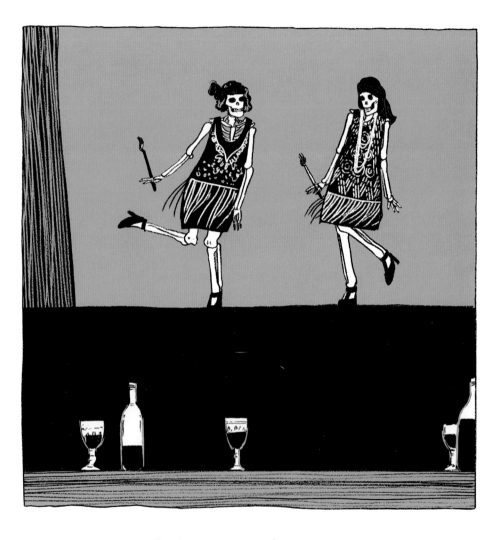

Radium made some flappers glow.
Tinted outfits they loved to show.
But while it made girls shine like gold,
it killed them before they got old.

Radium

Pity the poor radium girls, who only wanted to shine. In the 1920s, radium was used on watch dials to make them glow in the dark. Young women factory workers, who definitely did not know that overexposure to radium causes cancer, painted on the radium by hand. Lacking such knowledge, the girls not only licked their radium-covered paintbrushes as they worked to give them fine points, they also manicured their fingernails with the substance. Some also applied streaks of it to their dress buttons before they went off to nightclubs, where they would sparkle in the low light. But before long, the radium painters' teeth began to rot. When they went to the dentist to have their teeth pulled, some of their jawbones crumbled under the pressure. The condition was called "radium jaw." [1] The radium leached into their bones, permanently weakening them. The women were plagued with tumors and bone marrow damage, and by 1927, fifty radium girls were dead.

Scarves

What could be cozier or more delightful than a scarf? Or so you might think, but in reality, every time you put on a scarf, you might as well be wrapping a snake around your neck. Just look at what happened to poor Isadora Duncan. On a fall day in 1927, the famed American dancer donned her signature red scarf, which, according to one newspaper, "she had worn since she took up communism," [1] and went for a drive. But like the political movement, her scarf worked better in theory than in practice. As soon as Duncan began driving her convertible sports car, a breeze blew her massive scarf backward until it tangled on the rear wheel. Wrapped about her neck, it yanked her out of the car onto the street, where she died. "Affectations," Gertrude Stein quipped upon hearing the news, "can be dangerous." [2]

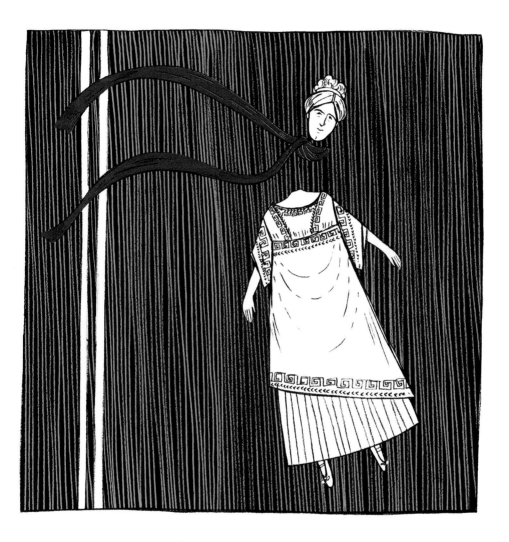

Isadora Duncan was Red.
Put on a scarf; popped off her head.
Fashion is silly, thought Stein.
It may tear your head from your spine.

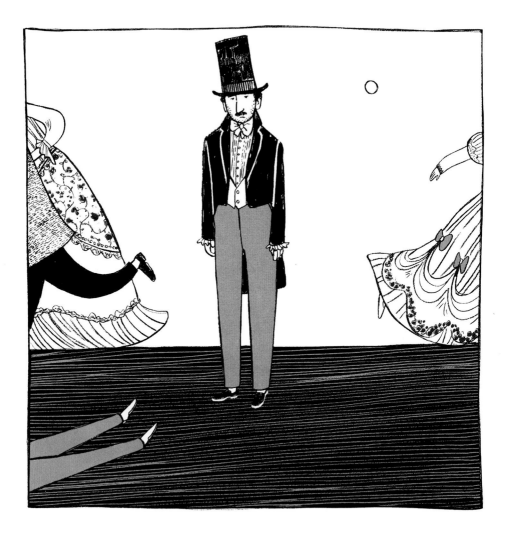

Hetherington debuted his hat,
the crowd went mad, a boy went splat.
Should've guessed from how tall he stood,
it'd be a crime to look that good.

Top Hats

"You might think of the top hat as the charming favorite accessory of cartoon millionaires such as Mr. Monopoly and Mr. Peanut, but like the origins of the Planters and Monopoly fortunes (for cartoons they seem vaguely evil) this adornment has a dark history. When London haberdasher John Hetherington first publicly debuted a top hat in 1797, onlookers were so terrified that it incited a riot. Women fainted, people screamed, and one young boy was trampled and left with a broken arm. Hetherington was later fined fifty pounds for "appearing on the public highway wearing upon his head a tall structure having a shining lustre and calculated to frighten timid people."[1] Top hats were outlawed in London for some time after. However, by 1860, across the Atlantic, Abraham Lincoln was wearing his to a much less riotous effect. Indeed, Carl Sandburg joked that the hat enhanced his safety as it made him "too tall a target" for the Confederate army.[2]

Viscose

Viscose was intended to be a less-flammable alternative to Chardonnet's artificial silk when it was developed in the early 1900s. But while it may have been less deadly for its wearers, it was not for its manufacturers. The material was made with carbon bisulphide, the fumes of which quickly drove workers insane. They began suffering from mania that prompted some factory owners to commission separate train cars so their workers would not harass other passengers while traveling. [1] Historian Alison Matthews David notes one factory went so far as to put bars on their windows so "workers, demented from carbon bisulphide exposure, would not jump out." [2] In addition to suffering from horrific bouts of insanity, exposure to carbon bisulphide also leads to Parkinson's disease. All in all, the flammable dresses of Chardonnet's design weren't so bad in comparison.

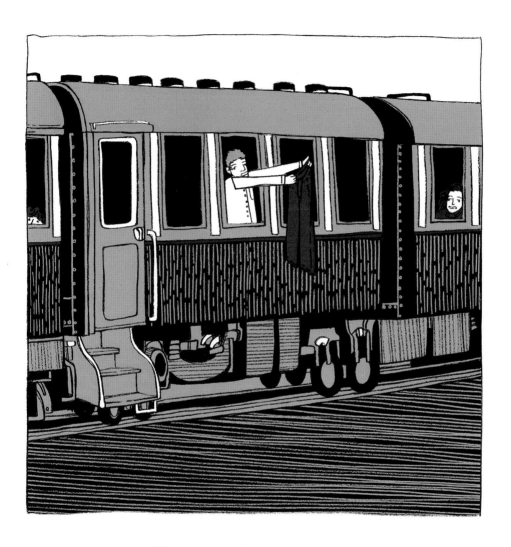

Viscose caught fire with far less ease
but brought its own kind of disease.
The poison fumes drove men insane.
You can't douse fires inside the brain.

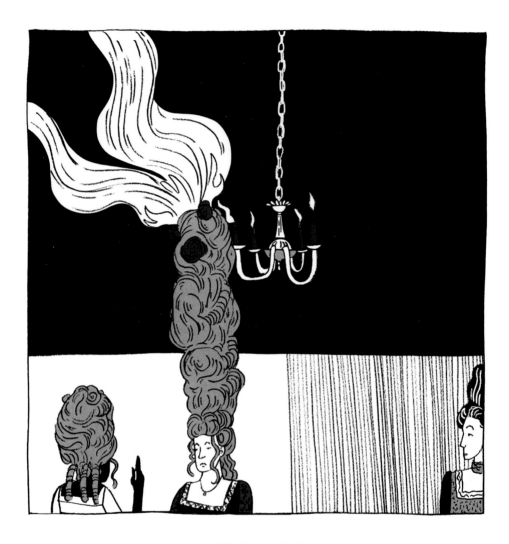

Animal fat kept wigs in place
so lovely hair could frame the face.
When candles set these wigs alight,
at least they killed the parasites.

Wigs

Blame Georgiana Cavendish, Duchess of Devonshire, for the wig trend that dominated the late 1700s. While wigs were already popular around the 1760s, fashion trendsetter Georgiana began wearing ones that were three feet high. [1] Society followed her lead, and it was soon unthinkable to appear in public without one's wig. Since animal fat was used to keep these wigs gleaming, they were highly combustible and had the potential to catch fire. [2] Even Georgiana was rumored to have attended a party where she bumped her wig against a chandelier, promptly setting it alight. [3] More repellent, and worrisome from a hygiene perspective, were the additional fashionable accessories the wigs required. Most wigs would be worn for weeks at a time, which meant that they would be crawling with lice. The solution was a special rod that allowed ladies to scratch their bewigged heads, presumably causing the bugs to swarm out most stylishly. [4] Author Summer Strevens recounts one urban legend about a woman at a party realizing that a mouse who had made a home inside her wig was gnawing on her skull. [5] Before long, Georgiana and her high-society copycats switched to adorning their hair with feathers, which had fewer disgusting and potentially fatal consequences.

Sources

Artificial Silk:

1. Allison Matthews David, *Fashion Victims: The Dangers of Dress Past and Present* (London: Bloomsbury, 2015), Kindle edition, loc 3342.
2. Ibid.

Asbestos:

1. "History of Asbestos," *The Mesothelioma Center*, last modified February 10, 2017, https://www.asbestos.com/asbestos/history/.
2. David. *Fashion Victims*, loc 3342.
3. "History of Asbestos." *The Mesothelioma Center.*
4. Ibid.
5. Rachel Reilly, "Woman, 66, killed by asbestos after washing her husband's overalls 40 years ago," *DailyMail.com*, last modified May 9, 2013, http://www.dailymail.co.uk/health/article-2318999/Woman-66-killed-asbestos-washing-husbands-overalls-40-years-ago.html.

Belladonna:

1. *Webster's New World College Dictionary*, 4th ed, (Houghton Mifflin Harcourt, 2010), s.v. "belladonna," https://www.collinsdictionary.com/dictionary/english/belladonna.
2. George Bacon Wood, *A Treatise on Therapeutics, and Pharmacology or Materia Medica* (Philadelphia: J. B. Lippincott and Co., 1856), 798.

Sources

Bras:

1. Hillary Busis, "Carrie Fisher Had Just One Request For Her Obituary," *Vanity Fair*, December 27, 2016, http://www.vanityfair.com/hollywood/2016/12/carrie-fisher-dies-strangled-by-bra-wishful-drinking.

2. Reuters, "Death By Wired Bras," *The New York Times,* October 28, 1999, http://www.nytimes.com/1999/10/28/world/death-by-wired-bras.html.

3. Olivia Chan, "Woman Saved By Her Bra After Being Struck by Lightning During a Storm," *DailyMail.com*, http://www.dailymail.co.uk/news/peoplesdaily/article-3226072/Woman-saved-bra-struck-lightning-storm.html.

Collars:

1. Fiona Macdonald, "Fashion victims: History's most dangerous trends," *BBC Culture*, June 24, 2015, http://www.bbc.com/culture/story/20150624-when-fashion-kills.

2. "Choked by His Collar," *The New York Times Article Archive,* September 15, 1888, http://query.nytimes.com/mem/archive-free/pdf?res=9907E3DC1F38E033A25756C1A96F9C94699FD7CF.

3. "Choked to Death by His Collar," *The New York Times Article Archive,* February 12, 1912, http://query.nytimes.com/mem/archive-free/pdf?res=9D0DEEDF1F31E233A25751C1A9649C946396D6CF.

Corsets:

1. Karen Bowman, *Corsets and Codpieces: A History of Outrageous Fashion, from Roman Times to the Modern Era* (New York: Skyhorse, 2016), Kindle edition, loc 1821.

2. Ibid.

3. Jackie Rosenhek, "Corset craze," *Doctor's Review,* January 2007, http://www.doctorsreview.com/history/jan07-medical-history/.

Sources

Crinolines:

1. Alison Gernsheim, *Victorian and Edwardian Fashion: A Photographic Survey* (London: Faber and Faber, 1963), 47.
2. Lucy Davies, "A visual history of crinolines - fashion's most magnificent disaster," *Lifestyle ‖ Fashion* (blog), Telegraph.co.uk, April 17, 2016, http://www.telegraph.co.uk/fashion/people/a-visual-history-of-crinolines---fashions-most-magnificent-disas/.
3. Bowman, *Corsets and Codpieces,* loc 1723.
4. "Burnt to Death," *Littell's Living Age* 70 (1861): 674.

Cuffs:

1. Suzannah Lipscomb, "10 dangerous things in Victorian/Edwardian homes," *BBC News Magazine*, December 16, 2013, http://www.bbc.com/news/uk-25259505.
2. David, *Fashion Victims,* loc 3342.
3. Charles Moore, *Plastic Ocean: How a Sea Captain's Chance Discovery Launched a Determined Quest to Save the Oceans* (New York: Penguin Random House, 2011), 28.

Felt:

1. John Cunha, Dr., "Mercury Poisoning," *MedicineNet,* 2017, http://www.medicinenet.com/script/main/art.asp?articlekey=81326.
2. David, *Fashion Victims,* loc 1039.
3. Ibid., loc 1218.

Fontange:

1. Victoria Sherrow, *Encyclopedia of Hair: A Cultural History* (Westport, CT: Greenwood, 2006), 134.
2. Summer Strevens, *Fashionably Fatal* (Amazon Digital Services, 2014), Kindle edition, loc 854-55.

Sources

Hair Dye:

1. Taylor Orci, "The Original 'Blonde Bombshell' Used Actual Bleach on Her Head," *The Atlantic*, February 23, 2013, https://www.theatlantic.com/health/archive/2013/02/the-original-blonde-bombshell-used-actual-bleach-on-her-head/273333/.

2. Susan Ohmer, *Glamour in a Golden Age: Movie Stars of the 1930s*, ed. Adrienne McLean (New Brunswick: Rutgers University Press, 2011), 190.

3. Orci, "The Original 'Blonde Bombshell.'"

High Heels:

1. William Kremer, "Why did men stop wearing high heels?" *BBC Magazine*, January 25, 2013, http://www.bbc.com/news/magazine-21151350.

2. Barbara Hoffman, "A new exhibit reveals the world's craziest heels," *New York Post*, September 7, 2014, http://nypost.com/2014/09/07/a-new-exhibit-reveals-the-worlds-craziest-heels/.

3. Amy G. Richter, "Churchill, Jennie Jerome," *American National Biography Online*, February 2000, http://www.anb.org/articles/20/20-01929.html.

Lead Makeup:

1. Stacy Conradt, "The Quick 10: The Fashions of Queen Elizabeth I," *Mental Floss* (blog), January 15, 2010, http://mentalfloss.com/article/23718/quick-10-fashions-queen-elizabeth-i.

2. Diane Mapes, "Suffering for beauty has ancient roots," *Health* (blog), NBCNews.com, January 11, 2008, http://www.nbcnews.com/id/22546056/ns/health/t/suffering-beauty-has-ancient-roots/#.WKTzvyMrITE.

3. Mike Rendell, *The Georgians in 100 Facts* (Gloucestershire: Amberly, 2015), item 31.

4. Emma Chambers, "Makeup And Lead Poisoning In The 18th Century," *University College London*, http://www.ucl.ac.uk/museums-static/objectretrieval/node/111.

Sources

Long Skirts:
1. "Septic Skirts," *New York Lancet* (June 2, 1900): 1601.
2. David, *Fashion Victims*, loc 697
3. Ibid., loc 709.

Lotus Feet:
1. Amanda Foreman, "Why Footbinding Persisted in China for a Millennium," *Smithsonian Magazine*, February 2015, http://www.smithsonianmag.com/history/why-footbinding-persisted-china-millennium-180953971/.
2. "TE.230: Bound foot of a Chinese woman 1862," *Queen Mary University of London*, http://www.qmul.ac.uk/pathologymuseum/specimens/items/133926.html.
3. Foreman, "Why Footbinding Persisted."

Muslin:
1. Tom Tierney, *Empire Fashions* (New York: Dover, 2001), 3.
2. Bowman, *Corsets and Codpieces*, loc 1503.
3. Strevens, *Fashionably Fatal*, loc 791.

Neckties:
1. Jamie Schram, "Suspect identified in necktie strangulation of rich widower," *New York Post*, February 7, 2017, http://nypost.com/2017/02/07/suspect-identified-in-necktie-strangulation-of-rich-widower/.
2. Carol Christian, "Paralyzed Houston man found strangled by his own tie," *Houston Chronicle*, last modified October 6, 2014, http://www.chron.com/houston/article/Death-by-necktie-Paralyzed-Houston-man-found-5804753.php.
3. Don Behm, "Teen strangled with necktie," *Journal Sentinel*, November 17, 2009, http://archive.jsonline.com/news/wisconsin/70301657.html.

Sources

Radium:

1. Denise Grady, "A Glow in the Dark, and a Lesson in Scientific Peril," *The New York Times*, October 6, 1998, http://www.nytimes.com/1998/10/06/science/a-glow-in-the-dark-and-a-lesson-in-scientific-peril.html?pagewanted=all.
2. Rebecca Hersher,"Mae Keane, One of the Last Radium Girls Dies At 107," NPR, December 28, 2014, http://www.npr.org/2014/12/28/373510029/saved-by-a-bad-taste-one-of-the-last-radium-girls-dies-at-107.

Scarves:

1. "Dancer Isadora Duncan is killed in car accident," *History.com*, http://www.history.com/this-day-in-history/dancer-isadora-duncan-is-killed-in-car-accident.
2. Strevens, *Fashionably Fatal*, loc 1021.

Top Hats:

1. Nigel Cawthorne, *The Ludicrous Laws of Old London* (Great Britain: Robinson, 2016), 65.
2. Stephen Carter, "Abraham Lincoln's Top Hat: The Inside Story," *Smithsonian Magazine*, November 2013, http://www.smithsonianmag.com/history/abraham-lincolns-top-hat-the-inside-story-3764960/#RxwLqCmdOfP4GmJ2.99.

Viscose:

1. David, *Fashion Victims*, loc 4061.
2. Ibid.

Sources

Wigs:

1. Stefan Kyriazis, "Deadly make-up, mouse-hair brows and lice-ridden wigs: The dirty lives of Georgian women," *Express*, August 1, 2014, http://www.express.co.uk/entertainment/books/494198/10-shocking-facts-about-Georgian-women.
2. Sherrow, *Encyclopedia of Hair*, 403.
3. Strevens, *Fashionably Fatal*, loc 838.
4. Kyriazis, "Deadly make-up."
5. Strevens, *Fashionably Fatal*, loc 838.

Killer fashion

Andrews McMeel Publishing
a division of Andrews McMeel Universal
1130 Walnut Street, Kansas City, Missouri 64106

www.andrewsmcmeel.com

17 18 19 20 21 SHO 10 9 8 7 6 5 4 3 2 1

ISBN: 9-781-4494-8713-3

Library of Congress Control Number: 2017936810

Editor: Allison Adler
Illustrator: Brenna Thummler
Art Director: Holly Swayne
Production Editor: Maureen Sullivan
Production Manager: Carol Coe

Attention: Schools and Businesses

Andrews McMeel books are available at quantity discounts with bulk purchase
for educational, business, or sales promotional use. For information, please e-mail
the Andrews McMeel Publishing Special Sales Department:
specialsales@amuniversal.com.